THE MIND IN SLEEP

Founded by C. K. Ogden

The International Library of Psychology

GENERAL PSYCHOLOGY
In 38 Volumes

THE MIND IN SLEEP

R F FORTUNE

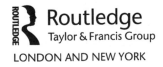

Routledge
Taylor & Francis Group

LONDON AND NEW YORK

First published in 1927 by
Kegan Paul, Trench, Trubner & Co., Ltd.
2 Park Square, Milton Park, Abingdon, Oxfordshire OX14 4RN
711 Third Avenue, New York, NY 10017

First issued in paperback 2014

Routledge is an imprint of the Taylor and Francis Group, an informa business

British Library Cataloguing in Publication Data
A CIP catalogue record for this book
is available from the British Library

The Mind in Sleep
ISBN 978-0415-21017-1
General Psychology: 38 Volumes
ISBN 0415-21129-8
The International Library of Psychology: 204 Volumes
ISBN 0415-19132-7

ISBN 13: 978-1-138-87523-4 (pbk)
ISBN 13: 978-0-415-21017-1 (hbk)

CONTENTS

FOREWORD

THE problem of the effect of a consciously held theory on dreams is one that requires some attempt at solution. There is a possibility that self-observation of dreaming may be nugatory if dreaming is greatly affected by conscious opinions regarding what may be expected to be found in it.

In the type of dream with which I shall deal in the following pages this possibility is at a minimum. It is a characteristic of the dreams with which I shall deal that they are in opposition, and in more or less direct variance, to consciously approved opinion. On these dreams conscious opinion has little, if any, effect. There is, however, another type of dream, a type that expresses conscious opinion in dramatic form ; and this type, in striking comparison with the type with which I am primarily concerned, is responsive to waking thought.

As particular proof of the freedom of the dreams

of my treatment from the danger which I have
indicated I may instance the dream that I have
named the dream of Stopes. It is Rivers' con-
tention that " the analyses of dreams which take
place under the dominant attitude of one who dis-
believes, or is supposed to disbelieve, in the
influence of sex will tend to give results in accordance with this attitude, or supposed attitude, of
the analyser." At the time of dreaming this
dream I had definitely rejected Freud's code of
sex symbolism. Nevertheless, far from my dream
conforming to my rejection of the code, remaining
in accordance with my conscious belief, it behaves
in a diametrically opposed manner, using one of
the least obvious sex symbols which Freud
mentions for a latent content most certainly
sexual. This freedom from consciously held
opinion is typical of the class of dreams which I
have studied.

Far from the formulation of a theory having
ordered my dreaming to pattern, it has apparently
had the reverse effect. The dreams on which I
have built my theory were all dreamt in 1923,
with the exception of the dream of Irises—at a

time when I had no certain opinion, no theory of my own, no attachment to Freud's theory, which they tend in some measure to confirm, and before Rivers' theory was published, or had reached New Zealand, a theory which they tend in great measure to confute. Since then I have noted but one dream in which this pattern has been repeated, the dream of Irises, which was not susceptible to such complete analysis as was necessary before it proved to be in conformity with my theory until six months after dreaming, and which, until then, I had thought was an exception. Since it is a characteristic of these dreams to be in violent opposition to consciously held opinion, it follows that, so far as a theory of dreams has influence on dreaming, such a theory should produce dreams which disprove it. Such an occurrence I have not noted ; and I think it is easily possible to exaggerate the influence of waking theory on dreams of the type under review.

The method of analysis was free association, not to all the elements of the dream, but to the elements felt to be most significant. This feeling practically invariably was discovered to be well founded.

Such free association took place immediately
after awakening. In the dream of the Library
Disorder the reconstruction of the submergent
was done some two years after dreaming, partly
by inference from the more obvious dreams of the
German Broil and the Library Vandalism. This
is not free association directly following the
dream—although the association " library disorder
—world disorder," the germ of the later inference,
did immediately follow dreaming. In the dreams
of Stopes and Irises the essential analysis was
obtained in a few minutes by free association—
but such free association was ineffective in the
recovery of very relevant parts of the latent content
which came back, in the one case two years after,
and in the other, six months after. With these
exceptions all the analysis was completed in each
case before breakfast, and usually before rising.
The three cases in which a later analysis was
admitted were cases where the earlier analysis had
already proceeded in the direction of the later-
discovered latent content, but had not penetrated
as deeply as subsequently became possible ; and
the added material was so relevant as to be taken

subjectively as proof of the accuracy of the earlier analysis. My impression was distinctly that it was not that the addition was doubtful, but that the forgetfulness had been pathological.

Five of the dreams of this book were originally published in the *Australasian Journal of Psychology and Philosophy*, for June, 1926, to the Editor of which I owe my thanks for permission to republish in this form. I have radically altered my earlier conclusions concerning envelopment, displacement and the place of affect in the dream. I now regard envelopment as confined to the dream of the Library Disorder, displacement as due to the continuance of repression towards the surrogate, and affect as a more variable factor than I had formerly shown from the evidence.

I owe my thanks to the several friends whose observations I have added to my own, whose objective spirit has allowed me in some cases to use very intimate matters for the furtherance of psychological science, a frankness without which the study of dreaming is impossible. I would instance particularly the dreamer of the Censer Dream.

I wish to thank also Dr. J. Drever, of Edinburgh, to whose kindly encouragement of a degree thesis this development of it is in great measure due, as to the University of New Zealand, who have furnished me with the necessary means to that end.

R. F. FORTUNE.

Emmanuel College, Cambridge,
  January 17th, 1927.

THE MIND IN SLEEP

I

SURROGATION

My chief purpose in this little book is to reveal a hitherto unobserved mechanism of a certain class of dreams arising from mental conflict. This class of dream may be roughly defined in terms first formulated by Graves: "when a person is in conflict between two selves, and one self is stronger than the other through waking life, the weaker side becomes victorious in the dream."[1] It must be understood that this is a very special class of dream and that many dreams within this class can only be included by a loose interpretation of the term "victorious." In many of these dreams the weaker side to the conflict evades repression during sleep in a very circuitous and symbolic manner and possesses the

[1] *The Meaning of Dreams*, by Robert Graves, p. 24.

field in disguise only. Nevertheless it is very convenient to divide all dreaming into four main classes, of one of which Graves' formula, widely interpreted, holds good.

Dreaming may be the dramatization of actual thought of waking life. It may be, again, a complete inversion of such thought. It may be so far removed from waking reality that explanation is impossible within the terms of present knowledge. Finally, it may be the release of a repressed tendency which has been repressed as the result of waking conflict. It is with this last class of dream that I propose to deal in the following pages, although I shall also touch lightly on the second class.

In these dreams where, more or less evasively, the dreamer is at the antipodes of his waking self, a repressed tendency finds release in a variety of ways. The first and most important method which I shall describe occurs where a repressed experience becomes confounded with a second experience symbolically similar but actually unrelated to it and differing from it in that it is not subjected to repression or, in some cases, to such intense repression. Between these two experiences there is always a community of affect. Two sets of experience come together and merge their separate identities so effectively that one of them formerly repressed shakes off its former repression with its former identity. These two experiences are cognitively but very remotely connected; but affectively they are closely related. It is literally as if a prisoner were to escape his warders by assuming the garments and counterfeiting the appearance of a visitor who was very like him in one particular, but only superficially like him in another.

The second method of evasion which I shall describe occurs when the straightforward release of one repressed tendency secures the release of another repressed tendency, not logically connected to it, but associated with it, although not by common affect, or feeling tone, as in the first method.

The third method of evasion is that of symbolic disguise. As this has been dealt with by other observers, and as my most reliable material falls more into the former two classes of evasive method, which I believe have not been described before, I shall not devote very much space to this third class. Certainty of correct analysis is very much more difficult to obtain in dealing with this type of dream.

Meanwhile I wish to raise two questions regarding the class of dreams that I shall describe. In these dreams an agnostic dreams with belief in Christianity, a pacifist with hatred of former enemy nations, an officer in the British Army dreams with a pacifist feeling towards a nation that he believed in fighting to the last, a devout Catholic dreams with complete agnosticism. Firstly, how is it that a weaker tendency can overcome a stronger, even evasively, in sleep when it cannot do so in waking life? Secondly, why should this dream revolution of attitude occur? To obtain an answer to these questions it is necessary to examine the actual evidence of dream inversion.

First it were best that I should define clearly the few technical terms that I shall find it impossible to avoid. Repression may be defined as the deliberate refusal to consider a certain line of

thought or action on account of its incompatibility
with an alternative preferred line of thought or
action.   The terms *censor* and *censorship* I shall
use to mean that side to a mental conflict which
is in the ascendant during waking.   The weaker
side to the conflict, the side repressed during
waking, I shall call the *submergent* in preference
to Freud's term which is derived from the
hypothesis that all dreams are wish-fulfilments.
The term *unconscious* I shall use to describe
mental states, cognitive and affective, which are
entirely foreign to the waking personality and of
which it is unaware, but which come into mental
activity during sleep.   I proceed now without
further delay to the evidence.

The Dream of the German Broil

In this dream I am debating the relative
advantages of a French and a German college.   It
is the time of the Great War and I am going
overseas to proceed with my studies.   Relatives
in France and relatives in Germany have invited
me to stay with them.   I pay a preliminary visit
of inspection to both colleges.   The French

B

college is on the flat in the heart of the town. The
German college is on the brow of a hill accessible
only by a steeply-inclined tram-line. I think
that the flat site is very convenient. On the other
hand, the hillside trams which lead to the German
college run very close to the home of my German
relatives. Finally, after some wavering, I decide
that, as France is our ally and Germany our enemy,
I shall go to the German college, and by this act
of magnanimity show my freedom from the narrow
nationalistic prejudices then convulsing the world.
I arrive at the home of my German relatives.
They receive me frigidly. X is staying with them
also. He completely ignores me. I know no
German, and no one makes any friendly advances.
I make some embarrassed remarks. One of
them is very foolish ; so X translates it derisively
and everyone laughs heartily at me. I go away
for a walk. Men lounging around the shop
verandahs quickly detect that I am an alien and an
enemy, and raise a hue and cry. I shake them
off after a rapid chase and arrive at the outskirts
of the town where the roads are lined with haw-
thorn hedges. I return home by unfrequented

ways after dusk.   My relatives and X ignore me
as before.   Next morning early I set out for the
German university college.   I board a tram and
proffer English money for my fare.   The conductor stops the car and orders me off.   I ascend
another car.   The conductor refuses my English
small change, eyes me with suspicion and refuses
to let me down at the college entrance.   Instead
he runs the car through the front doors and into
the interior of the building.   A gigantic wickerwork cage, shaped like a huge waste-paper basket,
is suspended about ten feet above the ground by
taut steel ropes attached to the rafters.   Into this
cage the conductor hurls me.   He then runs the
car away.   The car rails double back after it,
and I am left with no means of exit.   Various
officials come to inspect me there.   Some eye me
suspiciously, others derisively.   Some ask very
intimate questions.   After I have stayed aloft a
long time they release me and throw me
ignominiously from the front door of the building.

Immediately before retiring on the night of
this dream I had been reading an article in the
College magazine entitled, " This War—What

For?" It dealt with the diplomacy that nearly precipitated war between Britain and Turkey in 1922. It advocated a specific pacifism for each particular war in place of a vague "fair weather" pacifism that condemned war in the abstract, but made exceptions in individual cases. It advocated the purging of school histories from nationalistic bias, instancing an unfair attitude towards Germany in particular, and finished by quoting Romain Rolland: "To build higher and stronger, dominating the injustice and hatred of nations, the walls of that city wherein the souls of the whole world may assemble." This article had evoked my strong sympathy in almost every detail.

The dream opens with internationalism in the ascendant, as it had been during waking. Internationalism, the censor in this instance, expresses itself in the literal acceptation of the old taunt: "If you love your enemy, why don't you go to live with him?" I go to Germany rather than to France. The relatives in both countries are fictitious. Their only ground, in fact, is a very distant relative, my father's great-grandfather, with whose history I had only recently become acquainted at the time of dreaming, a Comte Debus, who fled the Revolution, married into a German family and emigrated to Australia. Yet, though I go to Germany in the dream, I still remain in my home town. The most striking fact of the dream is the coexistence of the belief that the colleges were in France and in Germany respectively, together with the imaging of them in the one locality, one in which I had lived some six years and more; a locality half the world away from Europe. There the dream college in Germany is situated. Its architecture and environs are those of an institution I once attended. The steeply-inclined tram-line runs between the town on the flat and the residential quarter on the hill where this institution is situated. X was, in my time, its Principal. The second great incongruity of the dream was the presence of X in the home of my German relatives. I had some reason to believe that he disapproved of pacifist activity. In the confusion of the German college and the college of my home town there was a complete absence of logical thought. I could never have made the association consciously.

I had a very keen hatred of the institution that I had attended; and I had been involved in two somewhat painful episodes with X. The gigantic wickerwork basket into which I was hurled in the dream is an exaggeration of the waste-paper basket in X's study, the scene of these troubles. My imprisonment in it, the butt of various objectionable officials is a good and true representation of my feeling of humiliation and distaste on these occasions, and my being hurled from the building is symbolic of the expulsion which at such times I felt could alone express their attitude towards me. The dream shows the affect of humiliation and hatred in a comparatively unrestrained, exaggerated and " all or none " form. My main reasons for objecting to the institution were the views that I held as to the inadequacy of no inconsiderable part of the lecturing, at which attendance was compulsory, not optional. Nevertheless I kept these views suppressed, and my feeling was complex, as despite the incidents in question I was very well and considerately treated by the staff. The dream does not show any evidence of this. There is release of repressed feeling in an exaggerated form that does some violence to my waking attitude.

The specific link between the representation of

> " the ghastly people of the realm of dream
> Mocking me. . . . "

and the article I had read the night before was probably the following passage from a history text-book for schools in India quoted in it:

> " The Germans are indeed a savage and a brutal race. In this War they have broken every law of God and every law of man. They say openly that solemn treaties are mere scraps of paper to be broken at any time they please; they kill their prisoners in cold blood, they torture those they do not kill; they murder women and children, toss them on the points of their swords and laugh at their screams of agony; they destroy churches and hospitals, they shoot doctors and nurses; they poison the wells and the streams and the air; they cut down the crops and the fruit trees; they lay waste the whole country as they go over it,

burning down the villages and leaving the towns heaps of smoking ruins. They are without religion, and in their cruel hearts there is no mercy, no pity, no kindness, no truth, no humour. They cannot be counted among civilized nations, and are indeed more like wild beasts than men."

In agreement with the writer of the article I had felt that this was untrue, unfair and prejudiced. But the citation of the passage awakened the hatred of Germany which I had once felt when I was a boy at school during the War. I had repressed this feeling while I was awake. I was unaware of its existence as an emotional reaction to the article. It remained unconscious, subterranean.

In the dream, however, the repressed hatred of Germany found symbolic expression. Early in the dream I continue the friendly overtures to Germany that I would believe in making in my waking thought. I even carry them to an extreme length by ignoring the War completely. As a natural enough consequence I am humiliated.

The affect of humiliation and powerless hatred which I felt in this dream was extraordinarily exaggerated and keen. From my real belief in the tolerable nature of German life I turn to my repressed belief in its intolerable nature. I go to Germany and find the people inhospitable and violent and I resent their conduct bitterly.[1] My own relatives refuse to speak to me. This repressed hatred finds expression by cloaking itself in a less repressed hatred of an institution I had once attended. I think it is fair to term my hatred of Germany unconscious, meaning by that term, unknown at the time of stimulation as a felt conscious experience. Then it may be said that an unconscious hatred finds expression by cloaking itself in a conscious hatred.

This dream throws some light on the theories of dreaming put forward by Freud and Rivers. According to Freud the dream is caused by the tension exerted on each other by two conflicting drives or impulses. One of these conflicting tendencies is the stronger and is named the

[1] In the year of this dream I acted as secretary (honorary) to a student body that was raising funds (by manual labour) for student relief in Germany.

censorship. During waking life it is able to exclude the weaker drive from consciousness. But during sleep the repressive force exerted by the censorship is lessened, though not abated, and the weaker drive can now come into consciousness, in a distorted form due to the impact upon it of the still active, though weakened, antagonistic force. This distorted expression of a weaker repressed tendency is known as the manifest content of the dream. The repressed material that finds distorted expression in the manifest content is known as the latent content. It is a cardinal point in Freud's theory that the dream is not to be taken at its face value, but that an underlying meaning is latent in its apparent triviality or absurdity.

This theory is fully confirmed by the dream under review. In it a deeply-repressed and unconscious hatred of Germany evades a pacifistic censorship in a symbolic disguise effected by merging its identity with a consciously-hated teaching institution, hated beneath repression that I had difficulty in sustaining. The incongruities in the dream are directly caused by this symbolic merging of two logically unrelated references. Freud's theory, however, is inadequate as a complete explanation of the dream. According to Freud the evasion of the censorship by the repressed insurgent tendency is due to a weakening of the power of the censorship in sleep. " The sleeping state makes dream formation possible by diminishing the endopsychic censor," he puts it. Actually we have no evidence of this hypothetical weakening of the censorship. In this dream, at least, we find a new mode of associative thinking whereby objects are connected, not by the logical relations of contiguity or cognitive similarity that obtain in waking thought, but rather by similarity of affect. This new method of association permits a novel relationship in which a repressed unconscious affect is associated with a relatively unrepressed conscious affect of a like quality and it is this new mode of association which allows a repressed affect to obtain release despite the continuance of the censorship. Freud has no knowledge of this mechanism of symbolism whereby a repressed experience merges with another experience less repressed, and so is made participant in the comparative freedom from repression of the latter; and he has no knowledge of the associative method of conjunction by community of affect which mediates this ingenious dream device. In consequence his account of a purely imaginary disguise devised by an insurgent repressed tendency to outwit a vigilant but occasionally sleepy censorship has provoked much opposition. The notion of a puritanical censor sternly insisting on a bevy of lascivious wishes donning Quaker garb before making their début in the dream has often been taken with humour rather than with entire seriousness. It has been dismissed far too easily; for, however allegorical an expression Freud may have given the facts, they remain and will continue to remain. Freud has unfortunately hidden his real discovery beneath a dogma that the dream is invariably a wish-fulfilment, that the repressed tendency that escapes in dreams can be nothing else than a repressed wish, and that in the majority of cases this wish is sexual.

It has been suggested to me that the dream of the German Broil is possibly a wish-fulfilment. I may have a repressed desire to suffer for my political convictions. The feeling that found vent in the dream was unconscious during waking. I have reconstructed it by inference only. Nor have I the means of denying what feelings I may entertain unconsciously. The subterranean persistence of long-discarded but formerly conscious modes of affective reaction in all their former intensity is one of the most striking phenomena of dreams. But it is bad scientific method to postulate unconscious feelings *ad hoc ;* and I do not believe that it is advisable to admit as unconscious any feeling that has not at some stage of development been fully conscious, pending later repression into unconsciousness. If it were otherwise, dream interpretation would vary with the mental vagaries of the interpreter. For the lack of some such postulate this variation has actually occurred between many of the opposed psychoanalytic circles. In the dream under review I do not consider that the wish-fulfilment theory is possibly applicable. It is plainly the release of repressed hatred and humiliation. I have never understood delight in victimization

personally or experienced any desire for such; and
the reference to hatred of Germany in the article
which provoked the dream as well as the unam-
biguity of my dislike for the teaching institution
and the humiliation I had of it, however much I
concealed it overtly, leave no shred of doubt in my
mind as to the only rational interpretation that
is possible.   It is a fundamental tenet of Freud's
most convinced followers that, until a wish-
fulfilment is discovered, preferably a sex wish-
fulfilment, and most preferably a sex wish-
fulfilment couched in complete physiological
detail, the analysis has not gone deep enough.
Why sex should always be associated with depth
is never clearly explained by them.   It appears
to be assumed that the dream regresses to infantile
experience deeply covered over, and again that
infantile experience most deeply repressed is at
the same time most certainly sexual.   I may say
in this connection that the theories of childhood
sexuality and invariable wish-fulfilment in children's dreams appear to be unfounded.   I have
the evidence of thirty dreams obtained from two
children aged five and six respectively.   I may

put this evidence into brief form by statistical expression, it being understood that the classification does violence to a few borderline cases. Twenty per cent. were wish-fulfilments, twenty-seven per cent. were conflicts between wishes and fears, mostly wish-frustrations. The remainder, constituting over fifty per cent. of the total number, were concerned mainly with pugnacity, rivalry and fear, fear predominating. These dreams were collected with the same care with which I collected my own, being recorded immediately after wakening. Not one of the thirty, collected from a boy and a girl, could possibly be interpreted in either the Oedipus or the Electra complex pattern by any fair-minded observer.

Rivers agrees with my position that the dream cannot be interpreted as a repressed wish-fulfilment. He agrees that the distinction between manifest and latent content is valuable and true. But he does not accept the theory of the symbolic evasion of the censorship in dreams. Rivers believes that the confused imagery of dreams may best be explained as regression to a lower more infantile level of thinking, postulating various mental levels on the analogy of the hierarchy of levels in the physiology of the nervous system. This postulation is admittedly hypothetical. I have shown that symbolism, together with affective association, may be a means of linking together two experiences, one repressed, one relatively unrepressed, with the result that one of them escapes repression in an evasive manner. The facts here are closer to Freud's theory of a symbolic evasion of the censorship than Rivers' proposed alternative to the hypothesis of the censorship and its evasion.

Before proceeding to the discussion of a second dream, I wish to recapitulate briefly the outline of the dream of the German Broil. The dream opened with an internationalistic or pacifistic gesture towards an enemy country—an expression of the censorship. The submergent hatred of that country found subsequent expression by merging and confounding it with an object of less repressed hatred which had played an extensive part in the dreamer's experience. There was a strong affect of humiliated hatred. The process whereby a more repressed experience becomes confounded with a less repressed experience of like affective content and so evades a censorship, is not an isolated mechanism. I shall require a name for the less repressed experience of like affect which serves to cloak the otherwise repressed submergent. This experience I propose to call the *surrogate* and the process of confounding submergent and surrogate by association through common affect I propose to term *surrogation*. Then it may be said that in the dream the submergent evades the censorship by surrogation. Using C to represent censorship, S to represent submergent and *s* to represent surrogate, the pattern of the dream is $C \underset{S}{S}$. This shorthand expression will prove valuable when somewhat more complex variations of these three factors appear.

In writing down a dream it is necessary to describe imagery verbally. In this verbal expression I have tried to preserve the atmosphere of the dream as closely as possible. Thus I did not comment on the coexistence of France and Germany in the one locality in the actual dream record, since in the dream no notice was taken of this,

c

and no exception was made to it.   The attention
paid to it was paid after wakening.   I fear, however, that I may have violated this rule in the
description " shaped like a huge waste-paper
basket."   That came with some illumination in a
half waking state subsequent to the dream, though
not to its recording.

The following dream conforms closely to the mechanism that I have already shown in the dream of the German Broil.

The Dream of the Library Vandalism

I have secretively let into the college library certain students that I thought I could trust. But they remove several window panes and smash the stained and frosted glass in other places. Then they set ladders up to the gaps and climb out through them on to the roof. After locking up the doors I meet in the passage two ladies, Professor K's daughter and Professor T's wife. As I pass down the stairs, Professor K, seated at the foot remarks loudly: " What's F been doing in the library at this time of the night? "

I awoke here, fearful, ran over the dream in my mind, and fell asleep before I could record it.

The same dream still continued when I awoke some hours later.

I am in the library and the glass is still unrepaired. Students are in, studying. But instead of supervising the room and keeping order, I am with the vandals of the former dream, dancing barefoot in a ring by the east table. Z distinctly says: " I had no reputation to lose any way; I didn't care what I did." The others express the same opinion. I feel my wretched position by contrast. Professor K comes up and says; " I want to see you outside, F." I reply: " In a moment when I put on my shoes and socks." I go out to look for him through passages, class-rooms, laboratories, but I find him nowhere.

I awoke, bathed in a cold perspiration, and noted quickened heart-beat and breathing. The evening of these two dreams I had thoughtlessly left on the lights of the library for over three quarters of an hour after closing time. My superior, the chief librarian, discovered this and came over in a rage. He succeeded in intimidating me somewhat, though I concealed my fear and put a somewhat careless face on it.

There was the danger that my carelessness might
be reported to the Professorial Board.   Nevertheless, I affected to pass the matter off as a trifle.
The censorship in this instance is my reluctance
to display fear and my appearing to minimize the
offence accordingly.

Professor K had not taken me to task over the
matter, although, as he was chairman of the
Library Board, he would have had to do so had it
been reported.   He had been associated with his
daughter in connection with the library once, and
once only.   Professor T's wife was then also
present.   That occasion was a Conversazione that
was held at the close of the meeting of the
Australasian Association for the Advancement of
Science in the summer vacation in January, 1923.
At this Conversazione which was managed by
Professor K, I had been (for a part of the time)
responsible for the care of the library until a very
much later hour than usual.   This was the only
occasion other than the inadvertent one on the
evening of the dream during my two years as
assistant librarian in the college, that the closing
hour had been later than 9.30 p.m.   I was new

to the work at the time of the Conversazione and was in some needless fear over the trust. My superior had protested strongly against the holding of the Conversazione in the library, and had wished that the books should be protected with wire-netting when his protest was overruled. This was not done, however, and his fears infected me somewhat. Particularly I had been warned that the bandsmen stationed in the library or the visitors might handle or displace books or periodicals. The submergent was the repressed fear evoked by the discovery of an unauthorized opening of the library till a later hour than usual. The less repressed surrogate was the solitary authorized opening of the library till a later hour than usual. In addition to the cognitive similarity between the more repressed submergent and the less repressed surrogate there was the similarity of affect, the fear in which both participate. The repressed fear of the unauthorized late opening, repressed by some hostility between myself and the chief librarian, was released by becoming confounded with a less repressed fear shared by both of us on a former occasion dating back several months when there had been an authorized late opening. The fear of the night before the dream I considered a weakness, the fear of the Conversazione night was rather that of conscientiousness. I certainly had a very hostile reaction towards the former fear, and no such repressive reaction towards the latter. It cannot be said in this case, however, that the submergent fear was unconscious. Nevertheless the affect of the dream is greatly exaggerated, and is different from that of my waking reaction, in which fear was in some measure overruled by resentment of the chief librarian's attitude, possibly in great measure, although I cannot gauge to what extent with any certainty.

The censorship in this case was my defence of my breach of the library regulations as being no serious matter. In the dream I allow students in after hours, as I, myself a student, had been in after hours. This expression of my actual defence, my taking apparently unimportant liberties with the regulations, leads to an expression of an unrestrained fear of serious consequences, complicated and allowed release by

cloaking itself in the guise of a former less
repressed fear marked clearly by the presence of
Miss K and Mrs. T in the manifest content.
Once released, the submergent fear in "all or
none" fashion proceeds to multiply imaginary
situations for its accentuated operation. The
pattern of the dream is again $C \mathcal{S}$.

It may be noted that the same dream continued
after a period of some hours of further sleep had
elapsed. A somewhat similar phenomenon is
recorded in the dream of Pharaoh, interpreted by
Joseph and recorded in the Old Testament.
Having awakened dreaming that seven lean kine ate
seven fat kine who had come up out of the Nile
before them, Pharaoh slept, and on wakening
again dreamt that seven lean ears of corn ate up
seven rank and good ears of corn. The connection between the dreams was patent to any
interpreter who knew that in the hieroglyphic
writing the cow was the sign for the earth,
agriculture and food, and that it was an animal
especially sacred to Isis, goddess of the fructifying
earth who was also goddess of the moon and whose
representation in the hieroglyphic script was the

sign for the year. Both dreams referred to a succession of harvests, the former referring directly to the Nile floods.

This reference of different dreams of the one night to the same content has been noted very frequently. According to Freud, Ernest Jones and other psycho-analysts, different dreams of the one night always refer to the same content. Rivers brings one case in support of this theory. I have a mass of evidence which I need not quote in detail, proving conclusively that all the dreams of the one night do not refer to the same content. In one case, six dreams were recorded on three spontaneous awakenings. The three dreams that came directly before the respective awakenings all referred to the same content and to an incident of the previous day. Dreams A and B were recorded at 5.45 a.m. Dreams C, D and E were remembered on a second awakening at 7.20 a.m. but E alone was recorded. Dream F was written down on the third awakening at 8 a.m. Then C and D, still vividly recalled, were written down. The six dreams are detailed, their manifest content alone occupying nearly six type-written pages of quarto.   B, E and F, coming immediately before each awakening, converge in the one content.   A, C and D have entirely different motives from B, E and F, A and D having a different motive from C.

I wish to point out that ordinary spontaneous waking appears normally to follow a dream which touches the most interesting or moving experience of the day or evening preceding.   This seems to differentiate dreams immediately preceding from dreams mediately preceding waking.   If waking occurs spontaneously more than once in the same night, convergence of content of the latest occurring dreams, those immediately approximate to waking (which is all that can be remembered except by exceptional observation) may follow from this fact and naturally lead to a belief that all the dreams of any given night have the same content.   This is true, however, only of dreams immediately preceding waking.   Even so, it is not invariable.

The following dream is one very far removed from waking, being separated from it by approximately twice its own content.   The absence of censorship and disguise is to be noted. As I shall show later the presence of the mechanism noted by Freud is peculiar to dreams occurring close upon waking, the censorship being essentially the return of waking consciousness upon a type of thought which actively resists such return.

Contamination Dream

I had come home and was sleeping in a living room, vaguely felt to be the library at home, but not looking like it. I was working very hard at a big table covered with papers. S was working at another table. It was very early in the morning. S yawned and said she could not work. I fluttered my papers and said in a very superior tone of voice, " Oh, I never get tired ; the longer I work the better work I can do." A man came in and said that henceforth we would have to work in the " hammock room." S said she could not work and suggested we go to bed to keep warm. I consented. She insisted in wrapping herself all up in a piece of mosquito netting, for " hygienic reasons," so that she would not get my breath. I reflected that the listerine was all gone, so perhaps that was just as well.

I was trying to catch a train.   I was driving a drag along a dirty road parallel to the railroad track.   It was a question of catching the train by reaching the crossing before the gates were put down.   S and little L were with me, sometimes riding on the drag, and sometimes slipping off and running behind, half hanging on.   Finally they both got off, little L saying viciously that she preferred to walk to being dragged through the dirt.   And I saw her foot scrape through some dry yellow horse manure.

The gates of the railroad crossing were down and a yellow cat had strayed inside.   I dashed in to save it and gathered it most affectionately into my arms, but it hunched away from me, scratching and struggling, so that I had to put it down, when it moved away and sat all in a hump with its back to me.

There was a group of miscellaneous people having breakfast, the kind of group one makes up travelling.   There were not enough dishes and the whole table was badly appointed.   Someone complained there were no little dishes for the jelly.   I tore off the corner of the bottom of a brown-paper bag and poured a spoonful of bright red jam on it. One woman said in great indignation, " Do you expect me to use that as a dish ? " I said, " No, I just meant it for a symbol and a declaration," and I lifted up the paper and showed a bright red stain on the wet white table cloth.

The general point of the dream is that the dreamer is regarded by various people as a contaminating influence. The incident of the listerine, a breath purifier, being used up was, in fact, true. The dreamer hated cats, a yellow cat having been her particular dislike all the previous winter. The dreamer's comment was: " that I should, contrary to custom and inclination, actually have risked my life to save that of a miserable yellow cat, and then that the cat should shrink from me in loathing is a very ironical circumstance." S was regarded as a woman who had failed in her work, and one of the women of the last scene was recognized as a very boring woman who compared every new place with others she had visited in far distant localities.

This dream represents one of the deepest excursions into a continuous train of dreaming that I possess ; and it affords confirmation of a conclusion that I had formed previously from a study of my own dreams concerning one of the most essential differences between the mind in waking and in sleeping. This conclusion is that in dreams association by common affect frequently supersedes association by contiguity and logical similarity. In this dream a number of apparently disconnected scenes are associated by common negative self-feeling, strongly projected. It is evident that affective association is a wider characteristic of dreams than surrogation, which is a particular application of the general tendency to the evasion of the censorship in dreams that occur close to waking, close to those returning waking attitudes that may be termed the censorship.

The fact that dream association is frequently association by community of affect rather than by logical contiguity or similarity has been noted before. John Abercrombie, writing in 1830, noted regarding dreams that they confused:

" Recent events and recent mental emotions mingled up into one continuous series or with each other, or with old events, by means of some feeling which had been in a greater or less degree allied to each of them, though in other respects they were entirely unconnected. . . . The only bond between these occurrences was that each of them gave rise to a similar kind of emotion, and the train was probably excited by some bodily feeling of uneasiness, perhaps an oppression of the stomach at the time when the dream occurred."[1]

" Entirely unconnected in other respects " is fairly applicable to the dream of the German Broil and to the Contamination dream. It is a slight over-statement if applied to the Library Vandalism dream.

Ribot, writing in 1900, said very acutely:

" Representations which have been accompanied by the same affective state tend henceforth to be associated; their affective similarity

---

[1] *Inquiries concerning the Intellectual Powers and the Investigation of Truth*, by John Abercrombie (Edinburgh, 1830), pp. 87-8.

forms a link between the separate representations. This is not the same as association
by contiguity, which is a repetition of the
experience, nor is it the same as association by
similarity in the intellectual sense. The states
of consciousness are linked, not because they
have previously occurred together, nor because
we perceive similarities between them, but
because they have a common affective tone.
Joy, sadness, love, hatred, surprise, boredom,
pride, fatigue, can each become a centre of
attraction, grouping representations of events
which are devoid of any intellectual inter-
connection, but which have the same emotional
tinge—joyful, melancholy, erotic, etc. *This
form of association is common in dreams* and in
reverie, that is to say, in states of mind where
the imagination works in perfect freedom."[1]

Baudouin's " Studies in Psycho-Analysis " is
primarily an attempt to explain dreams completely by Ribot's theory of association without

[1] *Essay on the Creative Imagination,* by Ribot (translated
Baron), pp. 87–8.

resort to Freud's theory. Drever notes that " similar feeling or 'affect' may bring together many strange bed-fellows from the point of view of waking conscious life."[1]

Freud and Rivers do not mention affective association. It is true that Freud states promisingly:—

> " The assumption is here made that the development of affect and the presentation content do not constitute such an indissoluble organic union as we are accustomed to think, but that the two parts may be, so to speak, soldered together in such a way that they may be detached from one another by means of analysis."[2]

The examples quoted in support, however, do not show association by common affect, but detachment of affect from a relevant image to an irrelevant image within the manifest content.

---

[1] *The Psychology of Everyday Life*, by J. Drever, footnote p. 144.

[2] *The Interpretation of Dreams*, by S. Freud (translated by A. A. Brill), p. 366.

D

III

ENVELOPMENT

THE dream that I shall bring under review in this chapter is one of very special and unusual interest. Early in the opening chapter of this book I quoted Graves' theoretical formulation:—

"When a person is in a conflict between two selves and one self is stronger than the other through waking life, the weaker side becomes victorious in the dream."

I then raised the question as to how it was possible that a weaker tendency should overcome a stronger. In the dream of the German Broil and the dream of the Library Vandalism it is evident that a weaker, and, throughout waking, a repressed tendency possesses the field, but only through that evasive process that I have termed surrogation. It would be truer of these dreams to state that the weaker side secures evasive release in the dream rather than that it becomes victorious. Nevertheless Graves' theory is literally true of many dreams. In the dream that follows the submergent actually stifles the opposition of the censorship, and emerges finally without evasion or distortion. A sudden variation in the strength of the censorship occurs within the manifest content itself. There is a sudden lapse of its power, and the submergent obtains direct expression following earlier indirect expression.

The Dream of the Library Disorder

In this dream I find myself in the library at my University College in deep theological altercation with the chief librarian. We move away towards the west end of the room to consult the library Bible. While our backs are turned a student jumps on a chair and delivers an address on the advantages of agnosticism to the users of the library who rapidly gather around him. I become infuriated at this and level a banana, revolver-fashion, at the group. They become intimidated and return to their work. When

order is restored I mount the chair in my turn and
deliver a counter-address on the great truth and
advantages of the Christian religion.

This dream nicely reverses my waking opinion.
Earlier in 1923 when the dream occurred, I had
moved at the College Debating Society " that
social progress has been retarded rather than
advanced by the Christian religion." That was
my sincere conviction. In that year I was
assistant librarian at the College and a part of my
duty was to keep order in the library. A disorder in the library was a hateful thing to me.
A mild disorder might occur once or twice a
term and require suppression. In the dream
agnosticism is inextricably confounded with this
abhorrent thing—the agnostic address is an
infringement of the library administration which
it was my duty to protect. Dreams often confuse
absurdly remote and different things. What
could be more remote than agnosticism and a riot
in a college library? Is it not utter foolishness to
confound them so? Let me take a more deter-
ministic standpoint. Here are two apparently
dissimilar things conjoined—why? My agnos-

ticism is ultimately based on the belief that the whole universe is an unguided and more or less chaotic disorder. In this dream I lose my agnosticism and turn to Christianity. To one who seriously entertains the hypothesis of an omnipotent Deity it is a hateful thing to be confronted with the fact of evil—the chaotic disorder of animate nature, one species preying on another, the cruelty of the selective fashioning of evolving life, and the final extinction of all life upon a frozen earth. It is all a vast, useless and unnecessary disorder and hateful—just as the imaginary library disorder of the dream would have been hateful had it occurred in actuality and not merely in imagination. In the dream I was deluded into thinking the library disorder was occurring in actuality. Accordingly it aroused my resentment. And because, from the orthodox Christian standpoint, the discordant universe that is the result of the viewpoint of physics and biology is hateful, and from the standpoint of an assistant librarian a disorder in a college library was hateful, the latter stood for the former in the manifest content. Hatred was the bond between

them and the fact that both were states of disorder.
I repress all belief in orthodox Christianity because
if I believe in a deliberate and foresighted creation
of the universe I must believe, for right or for
wrong, that its Creator is a Demon and hate Him
and His handicraft accordingly.   While waking
I do not indulge this hatred.   I regard the sum
of things impersonally.   I prefer to attribute evil
to blind force rather than to deliberate foresight.
I am too convinced an agnostic to do otherwise;
and it was two years afterwards before I saw that
I had really been venting a repressed sentiment
dependent upon a continued attachment to the
Christian faith in this dream.   For mark how
cunningly and adroitly it is vented!   It is confused and confounded with a far more open and
legitimate hatred of a library disorder, which is
a microcosm as it were, of the universal disorder.[1]
In the dream two experiences or sets of experiences
come together and merge their identity so
thoroughly that if one of them was previously
repressed it now shakes loose its former repression

---

[1] I use this term not of natural fact (as is obvious), but of
evaluation from a supernaturalistic viewpoint—disorder for
Omnipotent Benevolence.

with its former identity. It is literally as if a prisoner were to escape the warders by donning the garments and assuming the appearance of a visitor. These two merging experiences are slightly like each other (in the above dream both are states of *disorder*), but their main bond of union is the common affect or feeling in which they both participate. In the above dream both disorders are objects of hatred.

It may be objected that this is an unwarranted speculation read into the facts. I saw at first only that agnosticism, the censorship, in this case was deposed by becoming confounded with an object of hatred and so the submergent belief in Christianity found undisguised release. It was only after some time that I saw precisely why a library disorder appeared in the dream as the particular agency for deposing the censorship. The ground for my assumption of the hatred of the universal disorder as the submergent is that Christianity escapes repression undisguised at the close of the dream, and that if the library disorder be taken as symbolic the symbolism is very cognate and apposite to my waking views concerning that system of belief. So cognate is the symbolism that it may be not unfairly assumed that the sentiment which emerges undisguised at the close of the dream was active in the early more disguised stage of the dream. To allow some measure of verification for my assumption, I can only refer my reader to John Stuart Mill's essay entitled *Nature*. That influenced my belief more than any other written source.

In this dream there is, as before, a preliminary statement of the censorship—in this case agnosticism. The surrogate is the library disorder, the submergent the chaos presented by the biological and physical viewpoints, and the repressed hatred of it that was actually induced without repression under a former belief in a benevolent and omnipotent Deity. The repressed feeling is essentially that which has been finding recent legislative enactment in the southern United States. Its subterranean persistence is as remarkable to me as the persistence of my hatred of Germany. In both cases there had passed several years since either feeling had been conscious.

In the dream under review the submergent does

not appear in the manifest content confounded with the surrogate. It is a theoretical reconstruction in the earlier dreaming. The surrogate is confounded, however, with the censorship. The library disorder and the agnostic address are the one completely merged action. The pattern of the dream is not $C\,S$ as before, but $C\,S$. It follows that the submergent obtains unsymbolic, undistorted release when the surrogate is confounded with the censorship. In such a case it may be assumed that s carries the objectionable affect characteristic of S to C; *i.e.*, the censorship is infected with that very affect which causes the submergent to be repressed by it during waking. This disarming of the censorship, the lapse of its influence by infection with the affect of the submergent through its merging with the surrogate, I propose to call *envelopment*.

This process throws some obscurity on the cause of variations in the degree of symbolic evasion that occur in dreams in any particular case. In very many cases there appears to be no evasion whatever. This may be illustrated by the following dream:

The Dream of the Pike Attack

We were to storm a large house manned by German soldiery. We were outnumbered badly, but we had one advantage. The pikes that we carried were somewhat longer than the rifle and bayonet. I was concerned that my pike was not so sharp as my neighbour's. Then I found myself in a rush. In a minute I was in a room alone with my back to the wall facing eight or nine Germans. I felt a wave of fear sweep over me. But I killed them off and found myself outside gulping in the clear air.

The night before I had come from a pacifist address by Dr. M, with whose views in the main issue I was in agreement. The absence of symbolism is noteworthy when the dream is compared with the dream of the German Broil. Two explanations of the absence of symbolism in such dreams are always possible. In the first place waking may be sudden, when it may be conjectured there is not sufficient time for waking thought to come to grips with dreaming thought and to force modification upon it. In the second place envelopment of the censorship may have preceded the remembered part of the dream.

It is noteworthy that the dreams of the German Broil and the Pike Attack were both definitely stimulated by agreement with pacifist conclusions the night before dreaming. The subterranean continuance of past mental attitudes in all their former vigour is a very extraordinary phenomenon. It seems as if any accession in power or weight to the censorship must be followed by a complementary accession to the submergent. Otherwise the power of the submergent would remain stationary while that of the censorship grew, and the conflict would become progressively less acute. This does not happen. There appears to be an unconscious growth of repressed feeling parallel to the conscious growth of repressing feeling, a phenomenon which renders the facts of conversion comprehensible.

Unfortunately I have no record preserved of the events of the day before the dream of the Library Disorder. Every other dream that I have quoted is certainly stimulated by actual events and thought of the day or night before, and every dream, except the Contamination dream, which is removed from waking, is a reaction of resistance to the return of such waking thought by a violent expression of its opposite.

IV

Affect in the Dream and Displacement

I come now to dreams of a more personal nature than those already narrated, dreams characterized by strong repression, by the presence of displacement, complex symbolism and inappreciable affect.

I use this dream with some measure of reluctance. The content is not of an impersonal nature, and the necessary substitution of fictitious for real names destroys the actual record of the dream at its most crucial point. Some compromise must be made between scientific exactitude and the need for some reticence. I shall confine the substitution to two names only and I shall reproduce the likeness of the original as nearly as is possible. Let me call the school-boy character of the second scene of the dream by the assumed name of Stopes.

The Dream of Stopes

There are introductions made between three people. I am introduced to X. A train journey follows. I have arranged to meet X at the cross-roads. No one is there and I search everywhere distractedly. I am aware that X is not a real friend, but Musette, a woman character from Murger's " *Scènes de la Vie de Bohème*," while the other people of the introductions and train journey are other characters from the same book.

I then meet a school-girl from my old school, where the playgrounds are flooded out. I talk to her and then to B and Stopes and two other school-girls who are with them. I say that I have played cricket when the field was in worse condition than these fields (which are sheets of water). F and a lady and C pass, coming from a football match against a neighbouring school. C shouts: " Hullo, old eighteen fifties." Then everything and everyone disperses.

I am helping Mr. X, my old house-master to lop off branches in a pine tree.

The points I noted on waking were:

(1) I had not a remote suspicion that the dream had any personal origin or allusion. Until I had the analysis some ten minutes later the disguise was perfect. The lady of the first scene bore no outward resemblance to anyone of my acquaintance. She was merely a character from a book that I had read some months before.

(2) I knew B, F, C, and the school-girls (whose names I could give) quite well; whereas I had hardly ever spoken to Stopes. He had been several forms below mine. I barely knew him by sight. As I write now, over three years after dreaming this dream, his face is the only one of all the dream characters that I cannot recall. The others I recall with ease.

The extraordinary association of a stranger with others I knew so well aroused my curiosity the moment I began my analysis. I resolved to penetrate into the reason for this and thought it over till, in a flash, the disguise was laid bare. Let me suppose that the surname of the lady who was my very sincere friend was Marie. Let me suppose the book that I had lent from the college

E

library to a student the day before was " Married Love," by Marie Stopes. Stopes, the stranger, the unknown, appeared in a dream that was a dream of intimacies because there was a disguised wish-fulfilment effected by substituting Stopes for Marie, the real object of the dream, through the mediation of a book by Marie Stopes which I had handled the day before.

There the analysis ended at the time of dreaming. The book was not by Marie Stopes. It was by an author with a hyphenated name, and it dealt, among other things, with an aspect of birth-control. Marie was a lady I knew well; Stopes was a boy in a lower form at my old school, and was practically unknown to me. Two years after I suddenly remembered that I had been reading the " *Scènes de la Vie de Bohème* " at a time when I came to know that my feeling for the lady I have called Marie had been deeper than I had known. The gloom of the ending of that novel affected me as much as I could then be affected. I read into it what I felt to be a personal mischance. The extraordinary thing was that I should have forgotten this waking association of Marie with Musette (who had jilted Marcel somewhere about the last chapter) in analysing the dream. The association had been very definite and conscious. The repression directed against the dream thought kept this fact out of my mind for over two years, even after the disguise had been penetrated elsewhere. I may add that in the last scene, where I am lopping off pine branches, the symbolism has most certainly the significance that Freud attributes to it.[1] Not that I believe that the lopping off of branches always has this significance. I shall revert to this point, which is one of considerable importance, at a later stage.

I would never have made the association between the latter name of my friend and the former of the hyphenated names of the author of the book in question in my waking thought. In waking I did not normally think of Marie by that name, it being her surname ; nor is it a normal waking procedure to split a hyphenated name and use the former part of it independently. The

---

[1] Mr. X had been definitely associated in my mind in connection with sex conflict at puberty. I have no doubt of this point whatever.

relation of submergent and surrogate is as in the dreams cited previously. In connection with Marie sex was subject to heavy repression. In connection with Marie Stopes' book it was subject to no such repression, was consciously dwelt upon, and had, in fact, been discussed the day before.

The formality of the introduction at the beginning of the train journey may be taken as evidence of the first effect of the censorship. Where S, the submergent, represents Marie, s, the surrogate, Marie Stopes' book, and s' (Stopes) the appearance of the surrogate in disguise in the manifest content the structure of the dream may be represented:

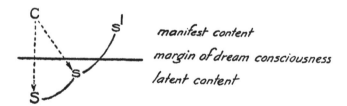

The most important image in the manifest content, s', does not appear in any conspicuous setting. On the contrary, it is comparatively hidden in a number of other images, apparently of equal importance. This process, where the image of the manifest content that has the greatest importance in connection with the latent content appears relatively inconspicuously in the manifest content, Freud has called displacement. Rivers and Morton Prince have denied the existence of this mechanism. Nevertheless it is apparent that it does exist, although not invariably.

Although it is clear that common affect had assembled the varying imagery of the dream, there was no conscious notice of affect in the dream on awakening—a striking contrast to the previous dreams cited, which were characterized by an extreme emotional quality. An erotically tinged French novel, a book dealing with birth-control and a symbol from one of Freud's most erotic pages were definitely used in a personal context and as symbols of a personal reference. No internal evidence for the water symbolism comparable to that which assures me of the sex latency of the lopping branches scene exists, but the tenor of the dream renders it not improbable that it represents the assimilation and use of a second Freudian symbol—despite a conscious

scepticism of a complete order on my part as to
the validity of Freud's theory.

I turn now to the dream of Irises.

The Dream of Irises

In this dream I am speaking at a public gather-
ing in favour of the Labour Party. Then I am
climbing, climbing, continually climbing a long
ladder. At the top I mount into a great cluster
of large red roses, very fragrant and extending
away a great distance on either side. I descend
the ladder. Half-way down is a long bed of
white lilies. I descend through them and come
at the foot of the ladder to a great bed of irises,
deep blue irises, extending, a solid mass of colour,
as far as I can see in either direction.

I awoke with a vague impression that I had
come from a dream of unusual beauty. Then
that riot of colour came back, first the irises, then
the lilies, then the roses and their fragrance,
heavy like that of the white China rose, and then
very vaguely, as from a great distance, the public
meeting where I had spoken in favour of the
Labour Party. Then I considered the dream as

a whole, or rather the word "irises" recurred
with such determined perseveration that I could
think of nothing else.   Then in a flash the dream
was as clear as the day.   Irises, irises—*flags*.
Red, white and blue flowers, and the alternative
name for the blue iris was flag!

Five days before the dream I had been staying
with some close acquaintances who were staunch
adherents of the Conservative Party.   An election
was approaching, and I became involved in a
political discussion in defence of the Labour
Party.   Labour leaders were charged with
accepting private moneys and with increasing
their own salaries.   I resorted to a *tu quoque*
argument, declaring that there was a far better
case to be made out against the disbursements to
the Royal Family as a national extravagance.   In
consequence I was accused of disloyalty with
great emotional heat.

The day before the dream I had revived this
episode by reading a Conservative attack on
Labour, wherein Labour was indicted as disloyal
and irreligious.   One commandment from the
decalogue of a Clydebank Socialist Sunday School

especially may have directly served to touch off the five days' old disagreement.

" Thou shalt not be a patriot, for a patriot is an international blackleg."

On the whole I agreed with that sentiment rather than the patriotism of " my country right or wrong " type, if not as an absolute statement, and felt that it was cognate to the Labour Party. In the dream I no longer agree. A mental upheaval takes place, and the Labour Party is closely associated with patriotism of the flag-displaying type.

In the dream the principles of the Labour Party regarding nationalism are the censorship. Ritualistic patriotism is the submergent. The censorship is briefly expressed at the beginning of the dream, as in the dream where I visit Germany; then, as before, it is abruptly reversed. The submergent, my repressed patriotism, so called, comes forth in a disguised flag of roses and lilies and irises.

There the analysis ceased at the time of dreaming. I believed that this dream was an exceptional case which showed evasion of the censorship without true surrogation. I could be reasonably certain, nevertheless, that I had the true interpretation, as the five days' old conflict had been a very severe and preoccupying one, the growing point of a difference of some standing concerning pacifism and militarism. The Freudian interpretation of ladder-climbing may have played some part, but I think a minor part, in obscuring a very relevant fact that came suddenly into my mind only just in time to allow me to send a footnote to the Australian Journal in which a preliminary article of mine on dreams was being published. Six months after the dream I suddenly saw its significance.

The night before the dream I had intended to go to a political meeting that was to be addressed by the new Conservative candidate for the Prime Ministership. I had tickets, but the necessity of proof-reading some typescript kept me from the meeting. Six months before, the former Premier, a strong Imperialist, had died. The school in which I was then teaching was dismissed. The headmaster was a Socialist and did not perform the customary weekly nationalistic exercise of having the children salute the flag. After all was cleared, we took a Union Jack from its locker and went to hoist it half-mast. Unfortunately there was no hoisting rope to the pole. Accordingly we resorted to the Fire Brigade Station opposite, carried the long Fire Brigade ladder to the school, and with some difficulty hoisted it. I climbed the ladder with the flag under one arm, with a wooden block and roofing nails in my disengaged hand, and nailed the flag half-mast.

Six months later I climbed a ladder into red roses, and down into white lilies and blue irises. The fact that the last image of the dream was fitted with the word *iris* rather than with the more revealing word *flag* on waking points to the influence of the censorship. The continued forgetfulness of the real ladder-climbing episode over a period of six months points to the continued influence of the censorship.

It is evident that the flag-hoisting was done, not to the memory of a good Imperialist, but to the memory of a political opponent who was dead. A more deeply repressed nationalistic feeling takes to itself a surrogate where the outward expression of nationalism was observed with mixed feelings, but with less repression of nationalism than any other occasion would allow. Repression was still directed towards the surrogate, however, for I had blamed myself keenly for a rash action I had committed when this Premier had been ready to plunge his people into war ; and I blamed his militarism for allowing my hotheadedness any opportunity. I regarded his death with mixed feelings, doing him honour grudgingly and tending to visit my own voluntary action on him. Consequently the surrogate is compelled to undergo a further process of distortion in order to evade the censorship. Where C is the Labour Party and pacifist censorship, S the repressed nationalism, s the less repressed nationalism on the Premier's death and s' the symbolic representation of s, the structure of the dream is as follows :

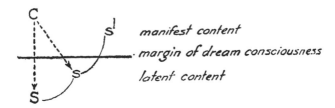

The most important image in the manifest content from the viewpoint of the latent content, the irises, does not stand out above the other images. Displacement of emphasis has again taken place.

There was no conscious notice of affect in the dream on waking, although the love of flowers, love of country motive is primarily one of affective association.

Considering the dream of Stopes and the dream of Irises together, we find :—

(1) Submergent and surrogate both kept repressed in the latent content.

(2) Forgetfulness of very relevant and obvious parts of the latent content until two years and six months after, respectively.

(3) Displacement in the manifest content.

(4) A punning relationship between the manifest content and the surrogate (in order not to reveal names I have not been able to reveal the full extent of this tendency in the dream of Stopes, where it is present in a further pun as ingenious as that of the flag in the dream of Irises).

(5) Affective connection of the imagery, without any consciously experienced affect in the manifest content.

These dreams are a very striking confirmation of Freud's and Rivers' agreed conclusion that affect in the dream varies inversely with the degree of distortion. The greater the tension between censorship and submergent, the greater the degree of symbolism adopted by the submergent, and the less release of affect in the manifest content. The contrast between the exaggerated and intense affect of the dreams of the German Broil and the Library Vandalism on the one hand and the absence of affect from the dreams of Stopes and Irises on the other hand is the most striking result that I have yet reached. The former two dreams are of the simple manifest pattern $C\mathcal{S}$, the latter two of the more derivative and complex manifest pattern $C\ s'$. The former two dreams may be regarded as the release of repressed affects, the latter two as the frustration of the release of repressed affects. The dream of the Library Disorder is an aberrant form, where the release of repressed affect is followed by the release of its

repressed cognitive content. The more success-
ful the censorship the less the release of repressed
affect. These dreams are primarily a war
between censorship and censored affect.

Displacement appears to occur when repression
is so heavy as to keep both submergent and
surrogate in the latent content, and when a play
upon words connects the image of which displacement may be predicted to the surrogate
which it symbolizes. Forgetfulness of latent
content and displacement alike seem to be due to
strength of repression.

The censorship may keep neither surrogate nor
submergent out of the manifest content. When
this happens there is a great release of " all or
none " affect, but only a very indirect release of
any repressed cognitive content.

Again the censorship may keep submergent, but
not surrogate out of consciousness. When this
happens there is envelopment of the censorship,
its complete lapse and a direct unsymbolic release
of repressed cognitive content, surrogate and submergent coming into the manifest dream separately
and in sequence rather than in a state of fusion.

Finally, the censorship may keep both submergent and surrogate out of consciousness. When this happens there is displacement, difficulty in complete analysis, and no release of repressed affect.

I propose to extend the term surrogation to cover all the facts of this first possibility, the term envelopment to cover all the facts of the second possibility, and I propose to term the facts of the third possibility, *substitution*. Symbolically, surrogation may be represented by $C\,S$, envelopment by $C\,S$ and substitution by $C\,s'$. These symbols may be used to express a number of known facts regarding affect and the like in these very different types of dreams, variants nevertheless of the one underlying plan. This plan is that which I outlined in the third paragraph of this book—a repressed tendency finds release by becoming confounded with a second tendency symbolically similar, but actually unrelated to it, and differing from it in that it is not subjected to repression or rather, in most cases, to such heavy repression. Between these two tendencies there is always a community of affect.

Writing in 1867, the Marquis Hervey de Saint-Dénis described some very interesting experiments which he had conducted during sleep for the purpose of influencing his dreams. He had spread on his pillow, after he had slept some time, an essence with an odour which was associated for him with a time when he had lived in the mountainous locality of Vivarais, and, at the same time, another essence with which he had often scented his handkerchief when he was working in the studio of M.. D.., a well-known painter of the period.

In consequence he dreamt at one time when this was done that he was dining in the living room of his former host in Vivarais with his host's family reunited to his own. Suddenly the door opened and M.. D.. was announced, the painter who had been his master. He arrived accompanied by an unmarried woman absolutely naked, whom the dreamer recognized as one of the most beautiful models that they had formerly painted at the studio. M.. D.. told how the carriage in which they were travelling together had been upset, and that they had come to ask hospitality.

Saint-Dénis draws a distinction between the memories of Vivarais and the memories of the studio on the one hand, and the ideas elaborated in the dream in order to weld the two memories, not logically connected, into some unity on the other. The ideas of his friends in Vivarais and of M.. D.. and his companion the model, he calls idées premières. The announcing of the new comers by a servant, the story of the overturned carriage and the like, he calls idées secondaires. In this dream he states that he has refrained from quoting many of the idées secondaires.

He then concludes that the cause of the extraordinary features of dreams is due often to the artificial rapprochement made between primary ideas by the secondary ideas.[1] Secondary ideas are taken as rational and satisfactory explanations of the conjunction of actually disconnected primary ideas during sleep, although to the waking mind the connection appears a transparent device.

I wish now to adopt this very fruitful distinction from Hervey de Saint-Dénis and to apply it to

[1] *Les Rêves et les moyens de les diriger.* by Hervey de Saint-Dénis (Paris, 1867), p. 382.

F

one of the dreams that I have cited. The primary ideas in the dream of the German Broil were the dreamer's college in his home town, and Germany. These primary ideas were as disconnected and as logically irrelevant as the scene of Vivarais and the scene of the atelier in the dream of the Marquis de Saint-Dénis. Instead of being connected by an external stimulus such as odours peculiar to each, however, they were connected by a common feeling tone—in the case cited, an affect of humiliated hatred. The secondary ideas were the refusal of English money by tram conductors, the chase of the alien through the streets, the coldness of the dreamer's German relatives— obviously devices that succeeded in making the home college appear as a German college rather than itself.

In the Contamination Dream there appears to have been no attempt at welding. The application is not so straightforward to dreams such as that of the Library Vandalism and that of Irises where there is an incidental likeness between sub- mergent and surrogate. Two occasions of late closing of the library, the death of a Premier and

the election speech of the man whose succession
to the Prime Ministership was reasonably sure—
such incidental likeness makes a closer connection
than is always found in dreams with association
by common affect, although it may be assumed
with reasonable safety that even here common
affect is the main associative factor.

The main point to be noted is that the welding
or secondary ideas are the more fantastic, more the
work of imagination.   It appears that the cognitive processes have been working in dreams
only to provide rationalizations that serve to
prevent the dreamer from knowing that the
connection between the parts of the dream is
irrational—as irrational in some dreams as if it
had been made by the experimental technique
devised by the Marquis Hervey de Saint-Dénis.

This fact is of some importance.   In these
dreams we have logically disconnected experiences
or situations thrust together in defiance of logic ;
but not entirely without order.   There is sometimes a slight and symbolic resemblance between
them from the cognitive viewpoint, such resemblance, for example, as is comparable to that used

in punning. More than this, both experiences evoke the same affect. This affect appears to have been effective in intermixing these logically separate experiences; for the result of the most overt evasion of the censorship is an exaggerated affectivity while, on the other hand, the result of the least effective evasion of the censorship, where disguise has succeeded only by becoming more covert, and where surrogate and submergent have been thrust down and kept in the latent content, is a diminished affect in the manifest dream. It is reasonable to suppose that the like affect, which, as a matter of mental history, is independently associated with both submergent and surrogate, is the effective agent in their association in the dream; for where submergent and surrogate appear in the manifest content, affect appears also; but where submergent and surrogate appear in the manifest content by symbolic delegation only, affect is not apparent there. It appears as if the affect of the repressed tendency were the prime rebel against the censorship, taking varied forms and guises upon itself in finding a vent, and exhausting itself in those cases where the censorship checks it in successive disguises and forces it into increasingly indirect channels. It appears that the complete repression of cognitive content would be theoretically possible if such cognitive content were not evocative of affects; for actually the repressed affect of any given repressed cognitive content will become free of its original content, transferring itself to a less repressed cognitive content of like affect, and so finding vent. The dream mechanisms that I have observed and described are well fitted to the theory that the emotions are " the prime movers of all human activity . . . and all the complex intellectual apparatus of the most highly developed mind is but a means towards their ends, is but the means by which these impulses seek their satisfactions." In dreaming mentality this theory becomes a definite fact. I do not consider that analogy from dreaming to waking thought is legitimate, however. Dream thought is distinctly *sui generis*.

The rôle of emotion in dreams has not been sufficiently observed by Freud, Rivers or other workers. The general claim I would make for my observation is that I have succeeded in demonstrating the essential similarity between dream and hysteria, a similarity that was suspected by Freud, but which his work on dreams failed to establish. If my reader will turn to the preliminary paper, the *Psychic Mechanism of Hysterical Phenomena*, published by Freud and Breuer in 1893, in which the discovery of the analytic cure of hysteria was first announced, and read it over in this connection, the likeness will become patent. There is the essentially similar conception of the hysterical symptom as a point of illogical attachment for an affect transferred from a not sufficiently " abreacted " trauma, and the theory of the cure by the direct, unrepressed " abreaction," or expression of emotion in its proper setting, instead of in the symbolic setting created by the detachment of the irrepressible affect. I had not read Freud and Breuer's paper, which was not readily accessible in New Zealand, until after my theory was independently evolved. In Freud's later work, much of which I had read, this earlier and, in my opinion, sounder conception was not present, as far as I discovered. As far as I can

tell, the parallel was reached independently.   It is
not in *Die Traumdeutung*, and it was not until I
read Freud and Breuer's theory of hysteria as
displacement of strangulated affect after my
preliminary publication that I realized that I had
brought the theory of dreams nearer to the
established theory of hysteria of 1893, demonstrating a closer likeness than had been observed
before.   The main difference is that Freud and
Breuer do not describe surrogation or the variants
of it.   They do not trace any association by community of affect between the trauma to which the
" strangulated " affect belongs and its hysterical
point of attachment.   The surrogate, if it exists in
hysteria, would tend to be difficult of detection,
probably being repressed out of the manifest
symptoms as it may be repressed out of the manifest dream by strength of repression.

The Biological Function of this Type of Dreaming

The mechanisms of surrogation, envelopment and substitution which I have described do not exhaust the possible methods by which a tendency of sleeping thought in active revolt against the return of waking thought can find play. The following two dreams illustrate the operation of the second method that I referred to early in my first chapter.

The Censer Dream

The dreamer is in a large house filled with his family and a number of people that he does not know. At one end of the front porch a Greek Catholic high mass is being celebrated. The ritual is unfamiliar and bizarre. There is a huge censer which the dreamer is told to light, igniting the white powder inside. After mass he is to cense the people.

He does not go to mass, being busy about the house, trying to fasten back a door which will not stay open. Suddenly he discovers that mass is over and that he has not been there to do the censing. He meets a somewhat heterodox attender at mass, and excuses himself for non-attendance on the plea of illness. The attender replies that he did the censing for the dreamer. He does not always go to church, but here he does. He likes the service. The priest and people preferred someone who was present through the mass, and who had entered into the spirit of it, to swing the censer rather than one rushing in right at the end.

The dreamer was of High-Church beliefs and was favourably disposed to the Anglo-Catholic movement. He was conscious, however, of a definite conflict between his religious beliefs including that of the sacramental nature of marriage and his loyalty to his wife on the one hand, and a desire to carry an extra-marital love affair beyond the bounds that his religious code and family loyalty imposed on the other. He had received a letter two days before the dream from the woman with whom he was in love reproaching him for his maintaining " le censeur " so rigidly and coldly. The letter ended " Vive le censeur! le censeur! le censeur! "

His family was agnostic and his early training had been entirely secular. His mature opinions led him to repress this early training. In the dream this repression is released. He fails in his religious duty of swinging the censer. The release of this repression, however, served as the release of the emotionally more important repression—he fails to maintain " le censeur " further. In this case there was a definite continuance of the non-religious attitude for some time after the dream. The sleeping thought was actually carried over into waking.

This dream shows that evasion of the censorship is not necessarily by affective association. Here there is not symbolism effected through the submergent becoming associated with a less repressed experience by community of affect. Here rather there is release of a repressed tendency towards agnosticism taking such an imaginary form that by a punning connection it serves as a symbolic release for a more deeply repressed sex tendency. This mechanism whereby the straight-forward release of one repressed tendency serves to release another more repressed tendency, recurs in the following dream.

Horse versus Motor-Car Dream

The dreamer is drunk; X, his friend, is drunk. The dreamer is in a horse-drawn trap going round the Basin Reserve. X is behind, sleeping huddled in the back of the trap. The dreamer is unable to drive. But the horse goes round the corners without guidance. The dreamer reflects how much better a horse and trap is than a motor-car when one is drunk. Near John Street a motor-car approaches sounding its horn. The dreamer takes up the reins which had fallen. The trap piles one wheel up on the foot-path. Here the dreamer awakens and hears a car passing outside his window, sounding its horn.

The day before the dream the dreamer had decided to repress his heavy drinking tendencies. He would get drunk no more. He had met W. An old woman driving slowly in a trap had passed them. The dreamer had commented on the obsolete use of horse traffic, condemning it roundly. W had suggested that it was in many ways preferable to motor conveyance, for instance it did not break down unexpectedly. The dreamer rejected W's defence as tenuous. He did not believe there was the slightest possibility of making a case against the immediate passing out of horse-drawn conveyance.

In the dream the repressed suggestion in favour of horse traffic evades the dreamer's antagonism by expressing itself in terms of the release of another repression. This device, which I propose to term *symbiotic association*, is essentially the same as that of the previous dream, except that here a resisted suggestion of lesser strength appears to avail itself of the escape of a stronger, instead of vice-versa, and one of the repressed tendencies is not repressed out of manifest consciousness. In yet other cases, as in the dream of the Pike Attack, the dream may possibly directly release a repressed feeling or suggestion with no device for out-manœuvring the censorship—unless, as is open to question, mere dramatization is such a device.   The following is of this dramatizing type.

The Dream of the Advanced Woman

The dreamer is walking with Z to whom she is engaged.   Suddenly she seizes the end of a sheet hanging down from a telegraph wire. Instantly the sheet travels away with her with great rapidity.   Soon she is far off, leaving Z far back in the distance.

The dreamer had decided to attend a University extension class in literature.   Mrs. A, her prospective mother-in-law, thought fit to object to this arrangement.   Her future daughter-in-law would get far ahead of her son and look down on him in consequence.   Advanced women made bad wives for ordinary husbands.   The dreamer who was a young lady with a fund of common sense, told Mrs. A that she thought her fears foolish, and that she did not intend to yield to them.   She would not get far ahead of Z.

In the dream Mrs. A's suggestion is given full effect despite the dreamer's waking dismissal of it.

I have described the unevasive dramatic release

of repressed material in dreams, evasion by surrogation, envelopment, substitution and symbiotic release by the close association of one
repression with another.   I wish now to mention
the existence of another method of evasion by
symbolism, where the manifest content has the
same relation to the submergent latent content
as the manifest content in the dream of Irises had
to the surrogate latent content.   The best example that I know is Rivers' Presidency Dream.
Rivers was in conflict between a desire to prosecute
his researches undisturbed and a desire to accept
the Presidency of the Royal Anthropological
Society.   He decided to reject the office.   He
dreamt that he was elected President, but his
election was made symbolically.   A man called
S. Poole was elected because Stanley Pool is the
centre of a great and complex system of rivers, and
because pools and rivers are alike in that both are
aggregations of water.   References to reading
matter in various places accounted for the particular form that the letters of the name assumed.

I wish now to turn to the problem of the
biological value of dreaming.   According to

Freud, the dream is always a wish-fulfilment. It banishes care and trouble and ensures untroubled sleep. Esther Griggs, who dreamt on the morning of January 4th, 1859, that her house was on fire, and who threw her baby out of a second-storey window while still asleep, and, under this impression, was guilty either of the murder of the baby, or of intent toward arson, for her dream was a wish-fulfilment. Fortunately the grand jury had no such belief. Nightmares are plainly not wish-fulfilments. Nor can it be said that nightmares protect sleep. Rivers put forward the opposite theory that dreaming is a lightening of sleep in order to enable speedy arousal in the event of the approach of marauding enemies or of other disturbance. Many dreams, however, seem to have little or no reference to external conditions prevailing during the night. Their originating cause is not a stimulus of the night so much as a repressed emotional reaction of the day, or days preceding, which would tend, if anything, to have an obstructing effect on a rapid cognizance of outward conditions.

In those lower animals which congregate in

groups or herds primitive suggestibility is over-
whelmingly strong.   The sight of a rabbit's
white tail bobbing sends every rabbit in the
vicinity to cover.   One bird rising raises a covey.
Sheep will follow a leader in jumping over an
obstacle removed immediately after the leader has
hurdled it.   Human groups, on the other hand,
often act differently.   There have been cases of a
steadfast minority firing on their own comrades in
retreat from the battlefield.   There have been
cases of conscientious objectors in war time.
Opposition to the group is a rare characteristic
even in man.   But it occurs far more often in
the human pack than in the wolf pack or in the
bee swarm.   Extreme flexibility to suggestion
fosters a strong group life, but leaves the individual
a social automaton, a cog in the social machine.
Extreme resistance to suggestibility makes the
individual solitary.   To make the individual more
than a cog in society, and at the same time to
avoid depriving him of the advantages of social
life entirely, it was necessary that the evolutionary
process should contain some means whereby
resistance to suggestion should operate without a

G

weakening of the normal power of suggestibility. This means is dreaming. Strictly speaking, man cannot resist the great mastering power of suggestion any more than the sheep, the wolf, the bee or the ant. Unlike the lower herd animals, however, he can defer the breakdown of his resistance till sleep. In the dream, suggestion that runs contrary to that general trend of suggestion acted upon during waking finds hallucinatory vent and secures emotional satisfaction. To make man suggestible at all involved making him suggestible to contrary and incompatible modes of thought and action, and it was necessary that contrary and dissociated modes of affect-charged thinking exist lest confusion and mental chaos result. One of these, association by intellectual and logical similarity or contiguity prevails during waking. The other non-logical association, symbolic or symbiotic association, or association by community of affect, prevails in sleep. Each mode of thought is only faintly impregnated with its complementary and opposite mode. The absurdity of dreams is in part the price man pays for being a herding animal. But it is only an absurd mode of thought from the point of view of an alien mode of thought.

It has long been recognized that the waking mind tends to become organized by grouping various emotional reactions about an object, or the idea of an object in its absence. Thus, the miser loves his treasures when he can touch and handle them, he fears for them when burglars break into his neighbour's house; he hates the thief if they are stolen from him; he envies anyone else the possession of similar valuables, and he covets such goods for himself. It must now be recognized that the dreaming mind is often organized differently. Various objects evoking the same emotion are grouped around that emotion. Thus the miser's fear of burglars, his fear of a Socialist Government and his fear of bulls, due to having been tossed by one when a boy, may come together in his dreams; as, to take a less hypothetical case, where R. L. Stevenson's schoolboy fear of examinations and fear of the Judgment Day used to coalesce in his dreams.[1]

---

[1] *A Chapter on Dreams from Across the Plains*, by R. L. Stevenson (London, 1920), p. 155.

The organization of emotions about an object is the normal mode of working of the waking mind. The organization of objects about an emotion, on the other hand, is a normal mode of working of the dreaming mind. I say "objects" advisedly, because the images of dreams are hallucinatory, appear as objects, and are reacted to emotionally as if they were objects. The waking unit of organization has been called the sentiment. The organizing activity of the mind during sleep is directed towards the breaking down of the sentiment, and the rebuilding of a new structure where the objects formerly at the core of their respective sentiments are regrouped about an emotional tendency that their sentiments have in common. This new structure I propose to call the constellation. Then sentiment and constellation may be defined as follows :

A sentiment is an organized system of emotional tendencies grouped about an object and the idea of an object.

A constellation is a collection of ideas perceived in hallucinatory fashion as objects, disrupted from the sentiments of which they form the core, and regrouped about an emotional tendency which their respective sentiments have in common.

Then the waking mind may be said to have the sentiment as its unit, whereas the dreaming mind often has the constellation. It is this radical difference in organization between the waking and the sleeping mind that assists in separating them so effectively, or rather, which is the device that the evolutionary process has perfected to keep incompatible suggestion separated. Close upon waking the constellation frequently takes a specialized form due to the impact of returning waking standards on dream thought in opposition. This modified constellation I propose to call the surrogate constellation. It may be defined as follows :

The surrogate constellation is formed by two ideas, perceived in hallucinatory fashion as objects, disrupted from the sentiments of which they form the core, and regrouped about an emotional tendency which their respective sentiments have in common, but which is more strongly repressed in one sentiment than in the other.

Frequently release from repression is secured

through the surrogate constellation, although, as I have shown, it may be secured in another manner than by any variant of affective association. Again repression may not be active, and release may be direct.

It must not be thought that all dreaming is of the type to which I have devoted most of these pages. These dreams occurred close upon normal progressive wakening when the influence of returning waking standards (which I have expressed by the term censorship) was brought to bear on dreaming thought violently in opposition to such standards. This violent opposition is, however, a wide-spread phenomenon. I may cite a few examples, if only to show that it is not an individual idiosyncrasy. Maury says that his dreams make him the victim of the very superstitions that he attacks when waking.[1] I, who, like Maury, know of no evidence for the existence of God, or of immortality, become a defender of Christianity in dreaming. Alice Meynell, on the other hand, a poet of deep religious feeling and sincerity, tells that :

[1] Quoted by Freud, *Interpretation of Dreams*, p. 61.

" I dreamt (no ' dream ' awake—a dream
    indeed)
A wrathful man was talking in the park:
' Where are the Higher Powers who know our
    need
And leave us in the dark?

There are no Higher Powers; there is no heart
    In God, no love '—his oratory here
Taking the paupers' and the cripples' part
    Was broken by a tear."[1]

After receiving a communication from the
Liberal Committee on Elections, of which he is a
member, Freud dreams that he receives a communication, in which he is treated as if he were
a member, from the Social Democratic Committee.
Wittels, in his book, " Sigmund Freud," in dis-
cussing the split between Adler and Freud, states
that the resignation of Adler and nine of his
adherents was in part due to political influences.
Adler and his nine sympathizers were members of
the Social Democratic Party.   Dreaming, Freud

---

[1] *Later Poems,* by Alice Meynell, " In Sleep."   I am indebted
to Mr. Wilfred Meynell for permission to use this poem.

becomes a member of that Party.[1] Rivers was an officer in the R.A.M.C. in the late war and a man convinced that the war was just and should be fought to a finish. I who, though not a Quaker, share the Quaker belief in the uselessness and immorality of war, dream an intense hatred of Germany, whereas Rivers dreamt a liking for Germany.[2] Pear, after deciding to relinquish some projected work on the lines of Shelford Bidwell's investigations, dreams that he continues it.[3]

At one time I thought that this violent opposition of dreaming thought to waking thought could be adequately explained as the release of temporarily repressed, but ultimately irrepressible suggestion; and I have not yet qualified this explanation. The objection to its adequacy is that the suggestion in opposition to the censorship is sometimes provoked by the mere reception of suggestion in agreement with that of the

[1] *The Interpretation of Dreams*, by S. Freud (translated A. A. Brill), p. 140.
[2] *Conflict and Dream*, by W. H. R. Rivers, pp. 117–27, 165 et seq.
[3] *The Analysis of some Personal Dreams*, by T. H. Pear, in *The British Journal of Psychology*, vol. VI, pp. 292–302.

censorship. In such dreams as the dream of the Irises and the dream of the Advanced Woman the censorship was only stirred into activity in resistance to suggestion to the contrary. But there are many dreams like that of the Pike Attack, quoted, where stimulation of the censorship is of itself sufficient to call up suggestion to the contrary though the mind must needs regress many years to discover it. In these cases, it is not explained why such material has not been sufficiently " abreacted " long before, and in cases where " abreaction," or release of emotionally charged repressed material, has not taken place previously, it is not explained why this release should be delayed throughout the night's sleep until immediately before wakening.

Moreover, there is a class of dreams that displays an equally violent opposition to waking thought where no suggestion of such opposition has ever been received by the dreamer. For example, a man speaks in passing of increased drinking of alcoholic drinks leading, in his opinion, to an increase in the spread of venereal diseases. He dreams that one of the group to whom he had said this is speaking in a public hall and selling bottles of an amber-coloured fluid, which is a new scientific discovery that will cure venereal disease instantly and easily. It is necessary only to shake the bottle. On waking he did not understand the dream until his statement of the previous day was recalled for him, when he at once saw the significance of the amber fluid. The dream was far more circumstantial and detailed than my account shows, with a wealth of chemical and medical detail in the dream speech.

Again a man dreams that he is at a boxing performance. One boxer is knocked down, but just before he strikes the ground his opponent quickly hits him as he falls. The crowd about the ring applaud. It seems the thing to do, so the dreamer, not without resistance, claps his hands with them. The night before, news had come that two candidates in a political struggle had polled an equal number of votes. The Returning Officer, in such cases, is by unwritten law expected to record his vote in favour of a candidate who has held the seat in the previous session as against a new-comer. In this case he acted without precedent and against custom in precisely the opposite manner. The dreamer had not been influenced by any suggestion that this action was praiseworthy.

Again, a dreamer sees X sitting at a table very sparsely set, and eating very sparingly. Someone says that he is always abstemious. Then someone contends that X's published work is very slender, and of poor volume. The dreamer becomes indignant and defends him, saying that, even if his work is slender, it is like a few snowdrops in a field of buttercups. The dreamer explained this last image as being equivalent to cultivated flowers among weeds. It was taken from an acrostic of the evening before. In point of fact X had been discussed the night before as an example of the use of wealth to make research easy, to subsidize assistance, and to finally produce a great volume of communal work without the stamp of that individual craftsmanship which means a great deal in research. X was the opposite of abstemious in ordering reprints of his articles, the number being two thousand in one typical case.

In these dreams a real situation is inverted

without any suggestion to such effect having preceded the dream.[1]   None of the few dreams that I have been able to collect from deep sleep by artificial wakening (after three hours) display the characteristic of opposition to waking thought, and although negative evidence is practically worthless here, I am strongly inclined to believe that the release of suggestion in direct variance and opposition to all that is believed in waking thought, and the imaginative elaboration of such opposition where opposed suggestion cannot be enlisted from the past experience of the dreamer, is a phenomenon that occurs only close upon gradual, uninduced awakening, and is most probably the expression of the resistance of an impulse to sleep to the return of waking thought. I am prepared to accept Freud's view that the

---

[1] This type of dream has been worked out in detail by Dr. Maurice Nicoll in his book, *Dream Psychology*.   His cases, however, are from patients suffering from mental disorder in which the inversion of waking thought is in the direction of sane comment, and not vice-versa, as is found in the same order of dreams in more normal cases such as I have cited.   For this reason I am not prepared to agree with Dr. Nicoll that this class of dream has any function towards the sane direction of waking life (Jung) in the generality of its occurrence.   In all this type of dreaming, however, lies the seed of mental upheaval, conversion etc. in waking life.

distortion of dream imagery is to be correlated with a function of guarding sleep exerted by such dreams as occur close upon waking. I am not, however, prepared to accept Freud's view that the censorship is the active agent, guarding sleep against the unpleasant tendencies that would awaken the sleeper were they not driven into symbolic ambush. According to the view here put forward the censorship is the awakening factor, being nothing else than the return of thought of the day before, and varying with the events of the day, whereas the tendency in opposition is an attempt to stave off such return. The submergent, not the censorship, is, in my opinion, the guardian of sleep.

I wish now to revert to two points arising from the dream of Stopes which I did not wish to obtrude while my concern was to show its structural similarity with the dream of Irises. According to Freud, dreaming very frequently, if not invariably, regresses to an infantile content. If a recent content is also present, as invariably it is, it is present in an instrumental function only. The infantile content uses the recent content as a cloak in which to disguise itself, to work in its interest as a workman works for an entrepreneur. This is actually true of the relation between regressive and recent content in the dream of the German Broil and in the dream of the Library Disorder if " infantile " be reduced to " pubertal." In the dream of Stopes, however, a recent content employs an " infantile," or rather a pubertal content as its disguise, in direct reversal of Freud's theory. The concept of one content being used instrumentally by another of a different time-level is valuable and true, but the time relation is not fixed invariably as Freud believes.

The second point arises from my employment of a symbolism derived from Freud's book in a dream that was one of ingenious and complex symbolism. The dream of Stopes presents three separate scenes. I think it is possible that each scene presents an increase in the complexity of the symbolism, the first scene being almost a literal extract from actual conditions with a punning denotation to one image, the second having a double punning denotation to one image, and the third using the symbolism of an extract from Freud. This increase in the complexity of symbolism towards waking in dreams of separate scenes has been noted by Dr. MacCurdy.[1] It is plainly evidence in favour of my opinion that the censorship is the gradual return of waking consciousness, and that symbolism is a protective device adopted by a resistance to such return when the conflict has joined forces.[2] If symbolism were a means of securing the evasion of the censorship, it would be incomprehensible that Freud's code of symbolism could be used to express repressed or dissociated matter in conjunction with a complicated non-Freudian symbolism; for it might be urged that the evasion of the censorship is impossible in Freud's code of symbolism to any person whose censorship is well acquainted with the code[3]; and the fre-

---

[1] *The Psychology of Emotion*, by J. T. MacCurdy, p. 484 *et seq.*

[2] This view of a progressive increase in symbolic subtlety of reference towards waking plainly agrees with my view of more complex symbolism and diminished affect in dreams of stronger as compared with dreams of weaker censorship. The fact is interesting when it is recollected that Dr. Rivers ascribed the more complex symbolism and concomitant loss of affect in dreams with recovery in cases of the war neuroses to his instructions to cease repression. In my own dreams increased symbolism with diminished affect is undoubtedly due to strength of repression.

[3] I am indebted to Mr. W. T. Armstrong of Cambridge for this criticism.

quency with which such a code is used by patients and others who have been made conscious by familiarity with it might be held to be indicative that such dreams do not express repressed, but rather surface material. The fact that this is not so points to the falsity of the " evasive " theory of symbolism. I possess more evidence than I have presented in proof that the actual state of affairs is otherwise than that which is the corollary of Freud's theory of evasion. To go beyond my own dreams I may instance two cases, that I can warrant as if they were my own. I regret that I cannot quote the circumstances in detail. In the one case a once consciously known symbol was being used obsessionally, in the second case an equivalently known symbol was used in a dream. In both these cases the sequel was a pathological forgetting of the significance of the symbol, once well-known consciously. This loss of a memory from conscious thought, after its acquisition and use by unconscious thought is a phenomenon that shows genuinely dissociated material finding dreaming expression in a code of symbols com-municated by the direct suggestion of the psychoanalyst, in one case by myself, the symbolism being my individual one. In both cases the symbolism was used for material indubitably most strongly repressed, and, for the time, definitely dissociated. It is this mechanism that is the possible justification of Freud's code of symbolism, providing, as it appears to do, a symbolic language in which the dreams of patients may express the unconscious causes of their trouble in a manner readily understood by their medical adviser.

I have defined unconscious mental states as being those of which the waking personality is unaware, which are foreign to it, and thereby disabled from a potentiality of coming into awareness, but which come into mental activity during sleep. Of unconscious states, otherwise defined, it is impossible to say anything. But unconscious thought in my sense of the term is clearly demarcated from conscious thought by three main characteristics.

In the first place a form of punning association is used without any intent of humour and with an entirely serious connotation. Verbal similarity is the basis for the fusion of entirely unrelated

H

references which are equivalent linguistically. A censer is le censeur, an iris is the Union Jack, the Assistant Registrary of the University of Cambridge becomes a Registrar[1] of Births, Deaths and Marriages and performs his duties accordingly in the University Office.

In the second place there is a form of association that is not linguistic, but is closely allied. The similar outer form or husk of events is made the basis of association, although the inner content, meaning and motive are entirely dissimilar. These cases are readily susceptible to expression in terms of linguistic similarity. A disorder in a college library is the disorder of the evolutionary process, a late library opening is a different late library opening, a Premier's death is associated with his probable successor's election speech. Attributes of the one are given to the other, though they have but the husk in common. This giving of the attributes of one event to another I propose to term simulacral association.[2]

---

[1] In New Zealand the one and the same term, Registrar, is used of both offices.

[2] It is because simulacral association obtains in code-uninfluenced dreaming that a code of simulacral sex symbols

In the third place, a form of association by common feeling tone is employed. Emotional quality is the basis for the fusion of entirely unrelated references which possess an equivalent background of affect. Thought is canalized separately by fear, hate, negative self-feeling, tender emotion and the like. In unconscious thought instinct-linked affect is isolated and most clearly demonstrated.

Two of these forms of association are found separately, and also in conjunction. All three may be found conjoined. Simulacral association I have not found in separation from association by common affect. I do not include under simulacral association the expression of an abstract or non-material concept in material terms, as is found, for example, in the dream of the Advanced Woman, or in a dream where the breaking up of a family is expressed in terms of the breaking up of a boat at sea of which the father is the skipper, and which breaks into two pieces with one half of the family on one part and the other half on the other, the

grafts on to dream thought, grows and becomes one with it Freud's code is true to dream type-thinking, a fact unrecognized by his dialectical would-be confuters.

steersman by bad steering being held responsible,
and incurring the blame (the steersman being the
dreamer). Such a mechanism does occur
separately, but it is a simpler process than that of
simulacral association, and is distinct from it.

An attempt has been made, notably by Jung,
Rivers and McDougall, to explain dream symbolism as vestigial from a lower and less evolved
type of waking thought which it is thought
prevailed earlier in the history of the individual
and of the race.   This explanation has been held by
its exponents to oust Freud's theory of symbolism.

It is certainly true that the early life history of
the individual is conducted with a vividness of
imagery that fades in later life—except in dreaming.   It is almost certainly true that savage peoples think with a wealth of very particular and
concrete terms and show signs of vivid imagery
in recall and description.   It is true again that
such peoples rely on a form of causation that in
our view is non-scientific, magical, simulacral.
Nevertheless, so much admitted, the vestigial
theory is not an adequate explanation of dreams
in which linguistic association and association by

common affect occur. It has yet to be shown that an involved word play and association by common affect are characteristic of primitive mentality or of infantile mentality.

The theory under review also fails to take into account the existence of dreams in which two antagonistic mental attitudes are clearly evident in the manifest content, and in which the transition from the one, approved and acted upon during waking, to the other, disapproved and repressed during waking, is also a transition from direct to symbolic statement. It must be remembered again that simulacral association in infantile and primitive psychology is not undetachably connected with association by affect as in dreaming. Again it is a great obstacle to acceptance of the infantile character of vividness of imagery in dreaming that the theory asserting such an explanation does not show why infantile and primitive characteristics should be combined with non-infantile and non-primitive characteristics within the one matrix.

The theory of regressive form in dream symbolism was probably suggested by the observed fact of frequent regressive content. As the conclusion of an analysis of seventy unselected dreams of my own, I found, excluding five cases that fell doubtfully, that fifty-six kept entirely within a three years' recency limit, four included scenes between three and seven years back, while five went back to puberty or very close to it. If, as I believe, symbolism is not regressive form, so coming into line with regressive content, the question suggests itself whether regressive content comes into line with a neo-Freudian theory of symbolism.

One of the main conclusions that have been reached in this study is that the associative processes in dreaming are frequently directed and guided by affect. This affect is usually not complex, but is of the kind that it has been held is the mark of instinctive behaviour (McDougall). Hate, fear, tender emotion, negative self-feeling and the like associate imagery, derived from perceptual situations evoking such affect as a matter of mental history, but which is kept in a state of dissociation during waking for logical reasons.

Evidence has accumulated in recent years showing that many instinctive and affective reactions continue in a decerebrate animal, but not in a purely spinal animal. A mid-organ, the optic thalamus, is now generally regarded as the main seat of affective tone.[1] If these general conclusions are accepted, and if thought and nervous activity run parallel, as we have every indication to believe they do, it must be concluded that in dreaming some subcortical and supra-spinal organ, probably the optic thalamus, exercises a direction and a control over the cortex. In waking, it is generally recognized, the nervous system may be regarded as a hierarchy of levels in which each level controls those beneath it, and is controlled by those above. In sleep it is reasonably certain, if thought and neural activity run parallel, a lower level may, and very generally does, control a higher. The case for this is as strong as the case for psycho-physical parallelism.

Meanwhile it is a definite fact that association by common affect is a wider and more frequent

---

[1] See *Introduction to the Theory of Perception*, by J. H. Parsons (Cambridge, 1927), p. 18 *et seq.*, also p. 71 in particular.

phenomenon than association by common affect complicated by simulacral association.   This latter case appears to be definitely produced by the impact of returning control in the cortical levels on a stronger form of association produced with the cortex under the control of a sub-cortical affective centre, probably the optic thalamus. Dreams such as some that I have dealt with leave their observer with a keen sense of strong and full affective association with but a comparatively frail cognitive association thrown across, however much the degree of frailness may vary towards strength in varying dreams.   Such association always bridges a waking dissociation, on the maintenance of which logical thought depends.   The dream association is primarily affective, sometimes with a secondary association of a simulacral logic thrown across in addition, sometimes not.

From this general point of view a clearer aspect of the reason for the stimulation of repressed attitudes close upon waking becomes possible. It may be questioned why repressed material does not find release until just upon incipient wakening when the repressing forces of waking thought are stirring into renewed activity. Why should release not have occurred earlier in the night with the censorship more in abeyance than it is close on waking? It can hardly be answered that no dreaming occurs until that time without making a vast assumption. The question is almost insoluble on Freudian rather than on neo-Freudian lines. But if control of the cortex by a lower centre occurs in sleep and is disputed by the awakening of the cortex and the incipient reassertion of the waking and downward system of controls, the upward system of controls obtaining in sleep, in asserting itself against resistance, will naturally be occupied with the weakest points in the resistance, *i.e.*, the repressed and the regressive cortical " tracts " rather than those corresponding to the returning waking and repressing standards. The facts are:

(1) Censorship and symbolism connected with submergent in dreams where the associative processes are directed by affect (dreams of German Broil, Library Vandalism, Library Disorder, Irises).

(2) A frequent conjunction of regression and

association by common affect in which the regressive scenes (with many years between them historically) are grouped about a single affect they possess in common. The dream of Stopes is one of several such that I have, and is quite typical in this matter of all.

(3) Association by common affect existing in a distribution wider than that of the censorship-submergent-symbolism pattern and the regressively-connected-separate-scenes pattern (*e.g.*, Contamination dream).

It must be admitted that this mechanism does not appear to apply so clearly to straightforward conflict that takes place without surrogation (Rivers' Presidency dream, Censer dream, Horse and Motor-car dream) or to dreams where an inversion of an actual situation occurs without any repressed or regressive foundation for it (see pp. 94-5). In these dreams there is no overt evidence of any upward control resisting the downward control that is initiated with wakening. Nevertheless in so many dreams overt evidence of such upward control exists, and that in those same dreams where overt evidence of the downward censorship control also exists, that it may be assumed that the two factors appear covertly as well as overtly together, and as a hypothesis, that such a direction of nervous control exists, even where not plainly evident, and is the correlate of the various types of inversion of attitude or of fact, frequently attended by marked affect, which form the body of these observations. It may be assumed that the initial conflict between higher and lower neural centres stirs a secondary conflict within the higher centre which may possibly continue under its own impetus, its initiating cause being hidden further back in the dreaming mind than the waking memory can always reach. I do not wish to lay undue stress upon this hypothesis; but I believe it is legitimate to infer the conjunction of covert censorship and covert affective selection of submergent in cases that share the linguistic symbolism and general structural opposition to conscious thought characteristic of dreams in which censorship and affective selection of submergent appear overtly conjoined, and in which there can be little doubt of the mechanism involved.

INDEX